Both Sides of the Iron Gates

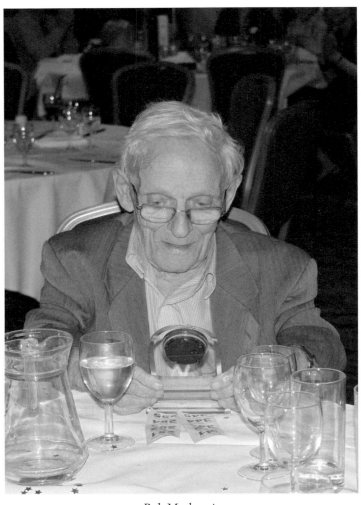
Bob Mackenzie
(1st September 1920–14th October 2012)
Bob received a Lifetime Achievement Award from the Restricted
Growth Association (RGA) in 2011.

Both Sides of the Iron Gates

BOB MACKENZIE

Born William Robert Mackenzie on 1st September 1920
in Newcastle Upon Tyne, England

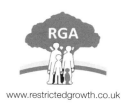

www.restrictedgrowth.co.uk

First published in the United Kingdom in 2014 by
The Restricted Growth Association

Book production by The Choir Press

ISBN 978-0-9930401-0-8

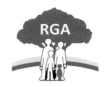

Contents

1

Early Years in Irons

LIFE IN NEWCASTLE was fairly good. My father worked in coal mining, as a skilled joiner, and with the mining rescue service.

One of the things I remember most was the daily routine at home in Newcastle. Before my father came home from the pit, Mother would fill several large pans with water and place them on the range, which was in the living room. Even if it was a warm day, the coal was loaded on to the fire. When Father arrived home he would remove his oilskin coat and leggings in the back yard. Then the large tin bath, which hung on the wall outside, would be brought in and placed in front of the range. We children were sent into the yard (or the bedroom if it was raining) and we were not allowed back into the room until he had had his bath and the water had been emptied – using the pans to carry the water to the sink, which was at one side of the range.

I spent a lot of my early years as an outpatient at the Newcastle Infirmary, in respect of my legs being very short and bowed. From the age of 3 years I had leg irons, for support and to supposedly strengthen and lengthen my legs. When it was time for me to start school, my parents insisted I went to the local infant school (and not to a special school) for which I will forever be grateful.

On one occasion, coming home from school with some of the boys, we had to pass an allotment which had a large bed of rhubarb, so of course we all went in and pulled a few sticks each. All of a sudden one lad shouted, "Run quick – the polis[1] are coming." All the lads were off like a shot, but I with my leg irons could only walk, stiff-legged, at a very slow pace. The bobby just gently and very slowly walked behind at a distance.

When I got home and went in, all seemed well. A little later came a hard and firm knock on the front door. Mother answered it and brought a bobby into the room. The policeman chatted to me for a while, telling me that I was a naughty boy, then wanted to know who the other boys were. I said I didn't know. He told my mother about the incident and also had a few strong words of advice to me. I promised him I would not do it again. The bobby thanked my mother and said, "Don't be too hard on the lad. After all, it is just the kind of mischief that boys get up to, but when we talk to them they seldom do it again." Then he went on his way.

No sooner had he shut the door than my mother gave me a good hiding and quite a few words. All was quiet for a while, then Dad came home and had his bath and meal. When it was cleared away, Mother said, "Willie, we had the polis here today: he's been taking rhubarb from the allotments." So I got another good hiding!

I also got into trouble at home, because sometimes I would venture down by the River Tyne (which was close by). The rowing boats used to go along with drag nets to catch fish. At odd times we would get a ride in front and sometimes, if lucky, we were given a fish to take home when we got back at the

---

[1] The police.

waterside to unload from the nets. My parents certainly enjoyed the fish, but as usual I got into trouble for being by the river!

Suddenly things started to become hard. The men from the pit went on strike, which went on for a very long time, and people were desperate for food. At school we were given soup and bread, I think by the Salvation Army. My father, in despair, left home to find work away from the pit. In September 1927, he sent for us all to settle in Birmingham, where he was now working. I can remember that day: as we were about to leave the house in Newcastle, my mother said, "You will not be wearing those irons any more," and off they went into the rubbish bin.

On arriving at Newcastle Central Station by taxi, I was over-whelmed by my new-found freedom. I was now able to walk without difficulty and bend my very short legs at the knee. Even my sister, now aged 5, and my brother, aged 2, seemed to enjoy the fun and were encouraging me to run about on the platform whilst waiting for the train.

What excitement – the first long train journey! I remember we stopped at York Station, where my mother met her sister Jennie and her family. It was the first time I had met them; they gave us some cake and sweets for the continuing journey. On we went in the train. In the afternoon we got to Chester-field and I could hardly believe my eyes – sitting in the compartment and looking out, I saw a twisted and leaning church spire. Having shouted and laughed, I was told all about it by a lady who came in at that station, which helped to occupy the last part of the journey.

We arrived at New Street Station with Father waiting on the platform. Once again there was a taxi to take us to our new home, which was in furnished rooms at Green Lane, Small Heath. We lived in the front room, which was neatly furnished with a sideboard, two high-backed easy chairs, and a table with four chairs. There were two bedrooms: Mother and Father in one; Betty, Ken and I in the other. We had two beds in our room, a washstand with a large jug of water, and a bowl for washing hands and face in the mornings. It was quite nice and comfortable.

We all got settled and my sister and I were taken to the local school, which was in Jenkin Street. I was now used to living without leg irons and, feeling a little superior, was told I had to look after my sister and take her to school. Walking from Green Lane to Jenkin Street meant I had to be careful, because we had to cross Coventry Road and be extra careful of tramcars. However all went well, thank heaven.

Then one Saturday afternoon I took my sister and brother to Small Heath (Victoria Park), where we played on the swings and roundabouts for some time. It was getting near tea-time and the other two wanted to go home, so I told them to start walking and that I would catch them up, as I wanted to have a last go on the helter-skelter. I set off to follow them, but when I got home they were not there. My mother and father went mad and sent me back out to look for them. I wandered around for about an hour but there was no sign, so back towards home I went. I was scared to go in, so I waited in Green Lane.

Then a police car came along the road, with two young children really enjoying themselves with the policemen. When my sister and brother had been reunited with Mother and Father, the policeman told the story of two children who had been found crying that they had lost their brother and didn't know the way home. They were taken to the police station in Tyseley. By feeding them and talking to my sister, the police still could not find out where they lived. But then Betty told them about school, so they were taken to Jenkin Street School. She said that she thought the way home was over where the trams were and from that they were gradually reunited with the family. Mother and Father were very thankful to the police for their efforts and understanding, but were not so happy with my story of events and I was dealt with in the usual way.

While we were at Green Lane, my father got a thing called a crystal set (which he said was a wireless set) and he could listen to music coming through the air with earphones attached to the set. The trouble was that only he could listen. Sometimes if one of us kids jumped about – or slammed a door while he was listening – he would get mad, as this meant that he had to fiddle about with the cat's whisker to re-tune it in.

2

On the Move

EARLY IN 1928 we moved to Hickman Road, Sparkbrook, which was a nice area. The house was fairly large, with a long hall with three large rooms and a scullery. The upstairs had three bedrooms, a bathroom and a toilet – with a further set of stairs up to two more rooms. As a family, we were well-off for the times: Father was working, Mother was nursing and looking after two or three very elderly ladies in the house. We had a large garden, with an apple tree and a pear tree, and with plenty of room for us three children to play.

My father fell out of work during 1929 and we moved into a very large house in Moseley Road, opposite the tram depot. There were a number of families living in the house and we were on the top floor. It was very different from Hickman Road.

At that time I was beginning to feel that something was wrong, as my mother and father were rowing. Then one morning I got out of bed and went to the living room. I pushed the door, but found the chain was on. I tried to put my hand around the door to undo it and could hear a hissing sound. After several tries, I went downstairs crying and told someone I could not get in. A man came upstairs, tried the door and then smashed it, went inside and turned off the gas. I was taken back into the bedroom, where I looked after my brother and two sisters. I think my mother was at work, nursing; she turned up a little later. It was all confusing to me.

The police came and also an ambulance to take my father away. Later that morning another ambulance came and took Mother, Betty, Ken, baby Jean (born the previous year) and myself to Western Road House (the workhouse).

A few weeks later the family was reunited, except for Jean, who had died of pneumonia. We went to live in a terrace in Sherbourne Road, Balsall Heath. It was a small house, with little in the way of lighting: in the living room there was an oil lamp on the table, in the bedroom were candles.

Our house had the brewhouse (wash house) right in front. On Mondays the women in the yard would be up very early, filling the boilers and lighting fires for the hot water, which they ladled into tubs. In went the clothes and they were churned about with a dolly. The clean clothes were hung out in the yard, on lines stretching from the houses to the wall. Sometimes we kids, coming home at dinner time, would run up the yard under all the washing lines and, on the odd occasion, would kick the prop. Then the women really let their tempers flare, arguing about whose child had let down their washing – which was now trailing along the brick yard.

We moved again, to rooms in Whitehead Road, Aston. I went to Albert Road School and, after the first week there, my mother and father were thinking of taking me away because they found out that the children had to buy their own pens, pencils and exercise books from the school. However, after talks with the school, I was allowed to stay and paid for basic items – this somehow kept the school somewhat select.

One of the items I remember at the school was the fire escape platform and the stairway from one of the classes on the upper floor. During hot weather the door was open and we would go down to the playground by this way, but on the odd occasion some boys would climb over the rail and slide down the supporting pipes, just like the fireman's pole. I did this once – in later life I have often wondered why, as I could have killed myself. It was a long way down and it was a very hard tar playground!

3

In the Jewellery Quarter

WE LEFT WHITEHEAD ROAD and moved to Warstone Lane, Hockley. The house was an attic-high back-to-back and right opposite the door and window was the cemetery, with tram cars passing by each way every few minutes. At the top of the hill was Joseph Chamberlain's Clock.

Inside the house, the front door led straight into the living room. In one corner was a black gas stove. In the other corner, near the entry wall, was a sink with a cold water tap. There was not much room; with a table, five chairs, and also a small cupboard (which stored the pots, pans, cups and plates on one side and the food on the other). My mother and father slept in the first bedroom. The attic had a double bed for me and my brother Ken, with a single for my sister Betty.

Up the entry was a small yard, with a row of twelve more attic-high back-to-back houses. One side got access from the entry next to our house, the other side from a little further up the road. Those houses had no water taps of their own, but got their water from one tap in the yard. The lavatories for us all were at the top of the courtyard (four houses having to share) and all the dustbins were in the same area. The smell at times was terrible.

When it rained the gutter in Warstone Lane used to be lined with pot plants, mainly aspidistras.

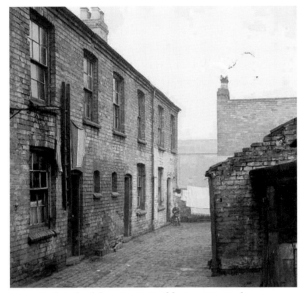

Back-to-back housing in Duddeston, Birmingham.
(Birmingham Lives Archive)

I went to St Paul's Church of England School in Legge Lane. When I started I was put in the bottom class for two days, then moved up to the next. After three weeks I moved up from Standard 2 to Standard 7, although I was only 10 years old. At that school you only moved up on ability; some 12 and 13-year-olds were still in Standards 2 and 3.

At times I sat up at night and watched the police march by in single file, with the back one dropping out to change over the shift. From my bedroom you could see a little way up Warstone Parade East and watch the policeman trying the locks and checking the windows by flashing the light he carried on his belt. At that time the police had put blue emergency boxes in certain areas of the jewellery quarter; a blue light flashed on top if the policeman was required, or if the policeman needed help it had a telephone inside with direct contact to Kenyon Street Police Station.

On Sundays, Betty, Ken and I went to church at St Paul's, which was known as the Jewellers' Church. After a short time I joined the choir. The one thing I do remember about being a choirboy, was that just before we moved into the church (having got dressed in cassock and surplice) the choirmaster used to give us each a small paperback Sexton Blake book to read during the sermon. These we hid under our surplices as we moved down the aisle to the choir stalls – it certainly stopped us fidgeting or talking.

St Paul's churchyard was also the only children's playground in the area and was called "Titty Bottle Park" by most children. There we played hide-and-seek among the gravestones. We had to make our own amusement and so we played games, either on our own or with others. We played marbles in the gutter; often we lost some down the suff (drain). We also flicked cigarette cards from our hands, trying to knock down other cards tilted against the wall. If you knocked one down, then you won that card and kept your own. Collecting cigarette cards and swapping them was a way of getting complete sets, usually 50 per set.

Another popular game was "Tip Cat". This involved a piece of wood – 1" square and 3" long – tapered to a point at each end (the "cat"), with another piece of wood to use as a bat. You placed the cat on the ground and struck the tapered end with the bat. The cat would then go up in the air and you used the bat to hit it as far as you could. There used to be many broken windows around, but it was never me! In the house the only game was draughts, which I played with my father, but he always won.

At odd times I would swap some cigarette cards for a magazine or comic. One was called 'The Wizard' and some of the stories were about men going to the moon and other planets. My father used to go mad at me, saying that it was a "load of rubbish" and "How could people get to the moon?"

I got myself a job as a messenger with Hodgetts and Son, a small jewellery place in Warstone Parade East which made brooches of dogs and birds. After school I would take the gold and silver moulds – which had been shaped and filed – to engravers (chasers), electro-polishers, diamond and stone-setters. Then at a later date I would collect them. At six o'clock I would also take a few small parcels to the post office, mostly to be sent by registered post. On Saturday mornings I would sweep the small workshop. All the sweepings and dust from the workshop were kept in a drum, which later went to the refiners to extract gold and silver dust.

For my average of twelve hours a week I was paid one shilling and sixpence (7½p in today's money). I gave my mother one shilling (5p) and the remainder I would spend by going to the Metropole Cinema, Snow Hill, on Saturday afternoon with Betty and Ken.

The cinema manager at that time was known to all the boys and girls as Uncle Wilfred. He used to come on to the stage and tell us about the next Saturday afternoon's programme. Sometimes we would also have competitions. On one occasion he asked us to guess the number attending that Saturday afternoon. During the week I wrote down the number I thought, then on the following Saturday my name was called out as one of the ten winners. The prize was to have tea with Uncle Wilfred after the film show, so I had to send Betty and Ken home. We all went up to the manager's office and inside was a small table laid out with jelly, blancmange, bread and butter, and plenty of cakes – it was wonderful. After tea he took us up to the projection room and told us all about it, in a simple way, without fancy technical terms. It was the first time I found out that the talking and music were on one side of the film, passing through a tiny screen on the side of the projector, and also that the lighting and curtains were controlled by the operator in that room. The tea and show-around took about an hour, then as we were about to leave we were given bags of sweets to take home.

My mother was nursing at Selly Oak Hospital on night duty six nights per week, which meant that she arrived home at about 7.30 am and got us children breakfasted and off to school. She would have a sleep till dinnertime, give us our dinner when we came home, then go back to bed when we returned to school. Later in the afternoon, when we returned home, I would go across to my job while Betty and Ken would stay in the house until Mother got up. She would then cook a meal ready for Father when he came home from work, so we all sat down at about 6.30 pm. Mother would be off to the hospital at 7.30 pm. She always looked neat in her uniform, with starched collar, cuffs and belt, and her white apron pinned under her coat.

But all was not well. Father was in and out of work a lot and I knew when out of work he would drink a lot, which meant that there were rows and upsets in which money was the arguing point. He also resented Mother working when he was on the dole. He would cause her to lose her job by telephoning the hospital and saying that she was not looking after her children. The rows got worse, even to the point where some of the crockery was being thrown about. Then I would try to get Betty and Ken out of the house and go for a walk. This was not always possible and often they were upset and cried.

One of the worst things to happen to Betty, who was a very bright girl at school, was when the school put her forward to take exams for George Dixon's Grammar School. She passed and was given a place at the school. Father would not let her go – just as he had done with me eighteen months previously – saying it would cost too much and also that the usual school leaving age was 14, but at grammar school it would be 16 years.

But still I used to be in trouble with both Mother and Father because of some of the words I had picked up, e.g. "miskin" (dustbin), "suff" (drain). "You're not to come home with those Brummie[2] words," they said.

When we needed coal I would have to go to the coal yard in Hingeston Street and get half a hundredweight, using one of their barrows to get it home. It took some pulling, up the hill of Warstone Lane. Then it had to be emptied down the cellar grating in front of the house. When you took the barrow back to the yard, you got the penny back that you had paid to use it.

On Mondays I would go to the butchers for twopence worth of bones and would also ask for some suet to be put with them. My mother would make soup with them, adding lentils and pearl barley. With the suet she would make dumplings and sometimes a suet pudding. She made enough to last two or

---

[2] Meaning 'from Birmingham'.

three days. One thing we never had was fresh milk; it was always tinned condensed milk, in tea or cocoa.

On the odd occasion, on Sundays, my mother would send me next door to Harris's shop with a cup and a penny to get jam for Sunday tea, which was a luxury. Harris's was a small grocery, sweets and tobacco shop, which was run by Mrs Harris, who was in her mid-fifties – rather fat, but very jovial and helpful to her customers.

4

Mother Makes a Decision

IT WAS A BEAUTIFUL, sunny morning in May 1933. My Mother had got me up rather early, about 7.00 am, and had told me to get dressed and not to disturb Betty or Ken, as she had something very important to tell me. I was intrigued to find out what it was, so wasted no time. Dashing downstairs into the living room, I noticed a large suitcase and a smaller one.

Mother said to me in a firm voice, "I have decided to leave him; I cannot stand it any longer. But don't worry, I have sorted things out. You, Betty and Ken are going to have a holiday together and in three weeks' time Betty and Ken will be going into the Middlemore Homes." To this I responded, "But doesn't that mean they will be sent to Australia or Canada?" I knew about the Middlemore Homes, because when we lived in Sherbourne Road we had some boys at school from the homes in St Lukes Road, and they used to tell us about some children who were sent to Australia, or Canada.

"Yes," Mother replied, "where they will get a better opportunity for the future."

"But what about me?"

"You cannot be accepted in the homes, as you would not be medically suitable to go overseas."

"What does that mean for me?"

Mother replied, "You will be able to stay at the holiday place till you are old enough to go to work, or if things turn out right I will be able to find a place where we will be able to live together. But please promise me you will not say anything to

Betty or Ken, only mention the holiday part. Now go and tell them to get up whilst I get something for breakfast."

I woke my brother and sister, telling them to hurry as we were going on holiday. The excited kids were up very quickly and soon downstairs. Breakfast was porridge, bread and jam. When we had all finished, Mother cleared up and tidied the living room. We all got on our coats and hats and walked up the road to the tram stop. After a little wait the tram came along. The conductor got off and lifted Ken on to the tram. Betty and I got on and Mother with the small case. The conductor put the large one under the stairway.

We arrived in town, by the art gallery and Big Brum[3] (which was as far as the tram went into town), and we all trooped off. Mother carried the large case, which was quite heavy. I carried the smaller one; even that was heavy for me. We walked through Victoria Square and into New Street. Right at the bottom we turned into the Bull Ring and stopped in front of St Martin's Church. Mother told us we had about a twenty-minute wait for the Midland Red bus. She gave Betty and Ken some sweets, which helped to quell the excitement they were showing.

The bus arrived and on we all went. I had noticed that on the front of the bus the sign was 'Bromsgrove'. It was getting very warm, so the bus windows were open. After nearly an hour the conductor came and told Mother that this was her stop, Lydiate Ash. Off we all got.

By the bus stop was a man with a push-bike. He greeted Mother and said hello to us kids; he appeared to be quite nice. He took the heavy case, placed it on the pedal of the bike and

---

[3] A clock in the centre of Birmingham.

secured it with some string. He also took the other case and, with one hand on the handlebars, he pushed the bike.

We went down a very long lane and then we came to a stile, which we were told to climb over. He had to loosen the case from the bike, pass it over to my Mother (who was already on the other side), then lift his bike over. We then walked down the side of a field (which he told us was wheat that would be turning colour very soon), then it was over another stile – with the same performance – into a very narrow lane. A short way down we came to a cottage and Mother said, "This is where you will be living for your holiday."

Once inside the cottage, the man – who said his name was Mr James – set to and filled a kettle from the pump outside. The kettle was put on the fire, which he stoked up and put on a few small pieces of coal. Tea was made and a few sandwiches. He told us we could have a look round outside, as he wanted to talk to Mother. We looked around: it was a fairly large garden with a spring at the bottom, very little in the way of grass and flowers, but plenty of vegetables. After a while we were called in and Mother told us to be good, to have a nice holiday, and that she would be back in three weeks' time. Then she kissed us all.

When Mother had gone, Mr James said he was going out to collect his wife from work. He would be about an hour and we were to stay in the garden till he got back. He then went into a shed and came out with a motorbike, which he pushed to the gate. I watched him kick-start it and, after a lot of tries, he got it going. Shutting the gate, we kids played around for a while. When we heard the motorbike returning down the lane, we ran and opened the gate. Mr James pushed the bike in and Mrs James followed on foot, having got off the pillion seat outside in the lane.

After a while Mrs James started to prepare a meal, and Betty was pleased to help. Ken and I just watched and talked. She told us that she worked at the laundry in Longbridge, then gave us a lot of information about the surrounding area and the walks we could do during the days. After the meal we were allowed to stay up till 9 pm! Then it was off to bed. The room was small, but we managed: Ken and I in a small double and Betty in a single bed. We were really enjoying ourselves.

In the morning we awoke to the sound of birds, which was certainly different to Warstone Lane – as was washing our hands and face at the pump outside, instead of at the sink in the living room. After the first week I was beginning to get the layout of the area, so we started venturing further. We had sandwiches and a bottle of water and stayed out most of the day. It was great fun!

The day arrived when my mother came to collect Betty and Ken. She told them they were going to a place that had donkeys and a big field to ride in. Mother talked with Mr James and I think some money was handed over. Mother kissed me goodbye and made off with Betty and Ken down the lane. Mr James said, "You're looking a bit sad, why?" I just burst into tears. After a while, I told him I knew that Betty and Ken were being put into the Middlemore Homes. He said it would not be for long.

After a few days, Mr James told me he had a letter from my father. He had to meet him the following evening and I was to go along as well. The next day I was on my own most of the time. Mr James brought his wife home as usual, on the motorbike. Just after tea, he told me to collect my things and put them into the small case. "We will take them just in case you are going home properly," he said. Off we went, with the case tied to the back of the bike and me on the pillion seat. I was told to hang on to Mr James's coat belt. It was my first ride on a motorbike and I was scared. We arrived at the Bournbrook Hotel, which was near the University. Mr James said, "Will you tell me when you see your father, as I have never seen him before?" Then I spotted my father and dashed up to him. Mr James followed and they started talking; I was told to go and stand by the motorbike.

Very soon the talk between my father and Mr James appeared to me to be an argument, which was getting nasty. Then Mr James came across to the motorbike, undid the case, handed it to me and said, "Go to your Father." He was off very quickly. I ran with the case to my father, who was walking away from me towards the entrance of the pub.

"What do you want?" he asked.

I told him that Mr James had gone.

"Well I suppose I will have to take you back to Warstone Lane," he said.

We got a tram into town and another from town to Joe Chamberlain's clock. I really thought I was going home, till we got to Mrs Harris's shop and went inside. She seemed very surprised to see us. Father said he wanted a quiet word with her. After a short discussion, Mrs Harris lifted the end of the counter, opened the small door and told me to go through to the living room at the back. She came in a few minutes later saying that my father had gone and I would be staying with them for the night. I was given some biscuits and a cup of tea, then shown upstairs to bed. Mrs Harris said, "Get some sleep, as you will be up early in the morning." I was wondering what was going on.

5

My Father's Plot

THE NEXT MORNING, Mrs Harris got me up early. After washing my face and hands, I went downstairs to where Mr and Mrs Harris were having breakfast. Mr Harris said, "Sit down, Son. Have some shredded wheat and bread and dripping." Mrs Harris gave me a cup of tea and said that my father would be coming soon.

He arrived at 8.00 am. While he talked to Mrs Harris, he told me to collect my things. He thanked Mrs Harris and she gave me a few sweets. Off we went, with my clothes in a small case. On the tram into town he told me that I was going to York and that things would be sorted out there. At New Street Station he took me down to the platform, putting me on the 9.00 am train. He gave me a letter with an address in York, also a single ticket. He said that the guard would tell me where to get off and that I only needed to ask for directions once I was outside the station. The train moved off. I did not realise, at the time, that I would never see my Father again.

We arrived at York and the people in the carriage helped me along the platform to the way out. Once outside, I walked a little way along the road. On the one side was a very steep, grassed slope with a wall along the top, built with large stone blocks. I then started to wonder how I would find the address on the letter.

I met some people talking, so bucked up courage and asked if they could put me right, showing them the envelope. One person was very helpful and, luckily for me, the address was just a couple of streets away. Having found Priory Road, which had lovely large Victorian style houses on both sides, I arrived at the house stated on the letter. I rang the bell. A maid in a black dress and small white pinafore answered the door. She asked what I wanted. I gave her the letter; she took it, told me to wait outside and closed the door. After about three or four minutes, I was beginning to wonder what was happening, as I could hear a commotion behind the door. Three men came to the door and one said, "Have you had your dinner?"

To which I replied, "No."

"Well, come along with us and we will get you something," they said.

We walked back up the road and came to a cafe. Once inside and sat at a table, they had a cup of tea each and I was given a meal of pie and potatoes – very nice. They talked away very quietly while I ate the meal, so I could not hear what was said. I was more interested in eating.

When the meal was over and the elder man had paid the bill, he collected a bag of cakes. We all left the cafe and I suddenly realised that we were going towards the railway station. When we did get to the station, they bought a single ticket to Birmingham and put me on the train – giving me the ticket, the bag of cakes, and also a few coppers: "For your tram fare at t'other end."

Arriving in Birmingham, I walked up New Street to Victoria Square, passed the art gallery, and caught the tram. It was well after nine when I arrived at Mrs Harris's shop. They were very surprised to see me: "We thought you had gone to where your mother was staying, now I expect you will have to stay the night. We will see what tomorrow brings – so off to bed." At a very much later date, I found out that my mother was at Priory Road when I called, but her sister's family had thought that my father was close at hand and they did not want him there.

I stayed with the Harris family, who were now wondering where my father was and why he had not contacted them. I started back to school. I also went to the jewellers and got my job back as a messenger. All seemed well, till one day I didn't feel well and Mrs Harris said, "You can't go to school today." A little later the School Board Man called at number 75, saying that Bobby was not at school that morning. The people who were now living there said they didn't know anything about it, but that there was a little lad named Bobby living at the shop next door. So the School Board Man came into Mrs Harris's shop to inquire. She told him that I was a little off colour and would be back at school the following day. She also told him about the circumstances which led to my being with them. He said he would have to report the matter to the Church and Education Department.

6

What Was Happening

ON 25TH SEPTEMBER 1933, when I was just 13, I was taken by Mrs Harris to a place in Wells Street. There in a room, sat at a table, was a man and two ladies. They had a few words with Mrs Harris. I could not hear what was being said.

I was called over to the table and the man said that, as my parents had abandoned me and the Harris family could not afford to look after me any longer, I would be better in the homes. He told Mrs Harris to take me to Summerhill Homes, on the Sandpits, by 3 o'clock that day.

Back home with the Harris family, I had dinner. They said that they were very sorry, but they had to obey the instruction. So at 2.30 pm I was washed and dressed, and off we went. It was not far: we walked down Warstone Lane, into Icknield Street, then turned left along Summerhill Road to the Terrace. Summerhill Homes was a large building with a highly polished brass plate on the entrance gate: "Children's Receiving Home".

The main front door was opened. Once inside, the matron took us all into a room. After a few words with Mrs Harris, a nurse came in and took me away to a bathroom. I was told to undress, as I was to have a bath. "Jump about lad, I don't have all day," she snapped. I was well scrubbed and then given their clothes to put on. They were not the best for fit; the short trousers were a little long (half way between my knees and ankles) and the shirt and jersey were too big, with arms that were far too long.

The nurse then took me down the corridor to a room and told me I was to stay in there. A little later she came back with a plate, on which were two thick slices of bread spread with syrup, and a mug of cocoa. It was tea-time, she said. I ate it and, after a while, she came in again saying it was bedtime – it was about 6 o'clock. She took me upstairs into a bedroom with two single beds. I was told to undress. "And put on that night-shirt," she snapped. I asked where the other boys and girls were and why I couldn't be with them. She replied, "You will join them when the doctor has seen you; that will be on Tuesday. Now get into bed."

I must admit, I cried. It was a very long night. With the window being open a little way, I could hear the trams running along the sandpits. I even went to the window for a while and just watched as they travelled along. Now and then I saw bright flashes, as the poles were running along the wires. For the next three days I was still alone in the room and after breakfast I was sent outside into the yard and told to play with a ball.

Tuesday arrived and I was quickly examined by the doctor, who told the matron that I could join the boys. The next day, after breakfast in the large dining hall (several long tables and benches, with boys at one end of the hall and girls at the other) I went to school inside the homes. There were two classrooms, one for 5-10 year-olds and the other for 10–13 year-olds. Both were mixed with boys and girls. It was different to ordinary schools, but the teacher, Miss Fry, was very nice and would not let the nurses interfere with her class.

A little while after tea-time we all went off to the bathroom (a bath every night), then to bed in a dormitory of eighteen beds. Some of the boys played up a bit and the nurse would try to quieten things down, but on one or two nights things got a bit out of hand; pillow fights used to take place and the lads would burst into song. It was not long before I learned the words:

> "There is a rotten home called Summerhill,
> where we get bread and scrape three times a day.
> Egg and bacon never seen, nor sugar in our tea.
> That's why we want to run away; far, far away."

This really got the nurses rattled. In fact, considering the number of children who went to Summerhill, there must be hundreds who knew and sang the song through the years.

7

The Iron Gates

ON 27TH OCTOBER 1933, I was moved – with nine other lads – from Summerhill Homes to Erdington Cottage Homes. After breakfast we were told that we were going to the Cottage Homes. A little later we all got into a van and about half an hour later we arrived at some very large ornate double gates in Fentham Road. This was the entrance to the Cottage Homes.

When the gates were opened, we moved just inside, trooped out from the van, and were ushered into the lodge.

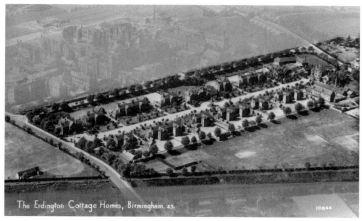

The Erdington Cottage Homes, Birmingham. 23.

Erdington Cottage Homes, Erdington, Birmingham
(*circa* 1930).

(Reproduced with permission from the Mary Evans / Peter Higginbotham Collection)

Once inside, the man who had opened the gates told us that we would be staying in the lodge for a few days, before being moved into a cottage. He was Father Lee and the lady who joined him was Mother Lee – we were to address her as "Mother".

Mrs Lee took over and we were all moved to the bathroom, told to remove our clothes while she filled two baths with hot and cold water, and in turn we were bathed. Then we were given clothes of the Cottage Homes. We went into the dayroom, sat down at a long table and had dinner of meat and mashed potatoes, followed by rice pudding. After the meal, we were told to fold our arms on the table and to rest our heads and keep quiet. That was the ritual during the eight days we stayed in the lodge. During our time at the lodge, we only went outside in the mornings – into a yard at the back.

On day three at the lodge, we were all examined by a doctor. I was checked over and then he told me that he would be seeing me again in about three weeks' time. On the eighth day, Mrs Lee told me I was being moved to Cottage No 16. Father Lee walked with me along the drive. On each side of the drive were Victorian built cottages, each fronted with grass and shrubs. Seven on the left for girls and nine on the right for boys – and ne'er shall they meet! Half way along the drive was a small tower with a chiming clock, surrounded by a neat lawn and floral beds, making an island. Further on the right we came to the last cottage, No 16.

The door was opened by an elderly woman. "Come on in, and who have we here?" she said.

Mr Lee said, "This is Bobby Mackenzie. Bob, this is your new Housemother, Mrs Griffiths." She looked me over and said, "We will have to alter those trousers and coat in a few days' time, so they will fit better." This pleased me.

I was taken into the large living room, which had two long tables with benches on each side. At the far end of the room was a big range, with a roaring fire between two ovens; this was the only means of cooking. Into the room came a rather tall and plump woman, aged about 30 years. Mother Griffiths said, "This is Miss Pegg. She will tell you what your duties will be. Every boy has to do a bit of work – you can start by putting out these knives and forks. Ten on that table and six on the other."

Just after 12 noon, the boys of the cottage came in from their schools: the older ones from Slade Road, the others from Osborne Road or the National. All came in the back way from the yard. After washing, we all sat down to dinner and said grace. Mrs Griffiths and Miss Pegg sat at one table with the six youngest boys. They had a tablecloth for their end of the table. I also noticed that if one of the boys was doing something wrong or talking at the table, Mother Griffiths' very stern look would be enough to correct matters. After the pudding, Miss Pegg told the boys who I was and said that I would be helping with the washing up or drying.

In the evening, at about 7.30 pm, it was time for bed. We went upstairs into one of the two dormitories, which each had eight beds. When we were all in bed, the lights were put out with a firm warning of "No talking." There were no internal toilets for the children, so a chamber pot was placed in the centre of the room.

On the following Monday morning, I was told to go with two of the boys to Slade Road School. Leaving the Homes at 8.30 am, it was a walk of about 15 to 20 minutes. After morning prayers, I was put into Mr Webb's class. Two days later Mr Webb said, "On Friday morning, Mackenzie, you will be going to woodwork class. I want you to tell the teacher that your first job is to make a stool, ten inches high. Then you will be able to rest your feet and your writing should improve." I completed the stool after three woodwork lessons with the help of the teacher. Whenever there was a change of classroom for other subjects, such as history, geography and science, Mr Webb made me take the stool with me – much to the amusement of the other boys.

Each morning, after prayers, the headmaster would say a few words on the interests of the day and also read out complaints from parents or local people. More often than not he would blame Cottage Home boys. We were told to stay behind, then he would ask us about the complaint. Never did a boy own up or tell on anyone, so we were all dealt with – one stroke of the cane on each hand. I think he suffered worse than us, as it must have tired him having to cane (on average) thirty boys! But generally schooling was good and we got along with the other lads.

However, as promised, the doctor sent for me. I went along to the infirmary, which was at the top end of the drive. It had two twenty-bed wards, one at each end of the building (one for boys and one for girls). Attached to each were three isolation wards and in between were the surgery and waiting room. All this was run by Sister Wilson, ably assisted by Nurse Oakley, Nurse James, and two junior nurses.

Sister Wilson took me in to see Dr Laverty. He asked a lot of questions relating to my legs, arms, height, and whether any other doctors had passed any comments that I could remember. I told him that school doctors always asked my mother about rickets, but that she had always said no. He then told me I would be X-rayed in a few weeks' time and that he intended to find out the problem.

Three weeks later, Miss Pegg told me at breakfast that I would not be going to school, as she was taking me to Selly Oak Hospital. It was a tram ride into town, a walk across to Navigation Street, and another tramcar along Bristol Road to Selly Oak. At the hospital we were taken to the X-ray department. They X-rayed both my hands and arms. We were then moved behind a screen while urgent cases were X-rayed. This was how most of the morning was spent: on the table, legs and feet X-rayed, then back behind the screen and so on. At dinner-time we went into a ward and had our meal with some of the walking patients. Then it was back to the X-ray department for a few more shots. Finally, it was the tram back to town and on to Erdington. During the whole day, Miss Pegg talked to me about school and asked about my earlier life. I then realised that she was human – and was concerned and dedicated to her job – not the terror I had been led to believe by the other boys.

A few days later, I was told to report to the infirmary after tea. Sister Wilson and Nurse Oakley were waiting for me. They said that Dr Laverty was there and was going to tell me about the X-rays. We went into the consulting room and he showed me some of the plates, although they did not convey much to me. He said to forget the word rickets and that it was Achondroplasia. He explained that what are called the "long bones" (i.e. the arms and legs) are much shorter than normal for me, but that the rest is normal. He told me that, at a guess, I would grow to between 4 foot 3 inches and 4 foot 6 inches. "Now! Listen carefully," Dr Laverty said. "You will be small, but most importantly you have nothing to worry about. You are healthy and as strong as an ox. If you use your brain, you will get along fine – so you have nothing to worry about."

I was now settled in at No 16 and found out that I was number three in line by age. My duties were to deck scrub and mop the large hall each morning before breakfast, and to wash up at tea-time. The lucky part was that one of the younger boys had to clean my shoes each day and, if they were not done properly, then I would make him do them again.

At the church, which was just across the drive from No 16, the Reverend Rhys talked to me and I let slip that I had sung in the choir at St Paul's, Hockley. He insisted that I join the choir. Mother Griffiths was not very pleased, as it meant choir practice two nights a week: "So don't think you will get out of your jobs and remember that, now you are in the choir, don't think you can join the band." The band practised three times a week.

On Sunday evenings, after church, the older children were allowed in the sitting room, where we would be able to play the wind-up gramophone. The popular tunes were 'In a Monastery Garden', 'The Laughing Policeman' and 'O For the Wings of a Dove' (sung by Ernest Lough).

All was going along fine. As the spring brought better weather, the boys were getting ready for the cricket season and I went along to the first practice match, which was to be played on the girls' playing field on the other side of Fentham Road. When I got there, the man who was organising the two teams looked at me and said, "You can't play – you're too small. But you can score. In fact, we will teach you to do the job properly. I will have a word with Mr Bryan, the superintendent." I found out that he was Mr Groom of Warwickshire, a player of some repute. The following week, I spent two days at the County Ground, Edgbaston, with the scorers in the pavilion and box. Boy was I looked after and spoilt!

So I became part of the cricket team and went with them to play schools and clubs around Birmingham and Sutton, which always ended up with an excellent tea.

The only thing I hated was when the barber, a Mr Paget, came every four weeks. He only ever used hand clippers and we all got pudding basin haircuts. We looked awful when he had finished.

During the summer, the senior boy had reached the age of 14 and was accepted as a bandboy in the army. He was a euphonium player, so he would be able to study music. That meant that I became senior boy, as the number 2 – Norman Hardwicke – was partially sighted and went to the special school for near blind children, in Whitehead Road, Aston. Norman and I got along well together and were friends. My duties took quite a leap: I had to flue and blacklead the large range every day (7 days a week), light the fire, then deck scrub the dining room with mop and bucket. And all was to be done before breakfast at 8.00 am. It was a rush to wash off the soot and grime in time for breakfast, and then to get to school.

During this time I received a letter from my sister, Betty, postmarked 'Gibraltar'. It told me all about the boat she was on and how she was enjoying the holiday, but had had to leave Ken behind. I was very upset, as I realised that she was on her way to Australia and that I might never see her again, and I could not even answer her letter. A week later another letter came from Betty, this time from Malta; then others from Alexandria, Aden, Ceylon, and Singapore, till eventually she arrived at Fremantle, Western Australia (W.A.). When she arrived at Fairbridge Farm School in Pinjarra, W.A., she and the other children found out that the so-called holiday was over and that there was no return trip. We kept writing to each other but, as it took six weeks for surface mail, letters crossed and caused confusion. She used to tell me about the beautiful weather and how the ground was mostly sandy, but that she was not happy about having to go about barefoot all the time.

I also used to get a letter from my mother about every three months. The postmark on the envelope I received was Deal in Kent, then it changed to Spalding in Lincolnshire, but there was always an envelope addressed to York for me to write back with, so I never knew where my mother was.

At the end of June we had the annual exams at school. These did not worry me, but just before the end of term the headmaster announced the results of the exams after morning prayers: "Top boy was Bobby Mackenzie." Then he put in a few extra words, "I am surprised that you have let a Cottage Homes boy beat you all." To this I shouted back in temper, "Why not? We are as good as everybody else." I was told to report to the head after assembly and got six of the best – three on each hand – for what he called being "cheeky and aggressive".

When I got back to the Homes, the Superintendent sent for me. He had been told of my outburst. He said that he understood, but that I should not have reacted that way.

"It is better to ignore those kinds of remarks. Away you go and forget it."

Mr and Mrs Bryan, the Superintendent and Matron, were wonderful, kind and understanding. They were certainly respected by the children and staff.

I was expecting to leave school at the August holidays, but I had to stay on until the end of October because my birthday was the day after August 31st.

The Cottage Homes took all the children over 7 years of age to Rhyl, for one week. There was tremendous excitement – marching to Gravelly Hill station and boarding the train especially for us. On arrival at Rhyl, we marched to a school a little way from the station. We all settled in and were fed. In the evening, we all had to make our own beds. We were given a mattress cover, which we filled with the straw that was piled in the corner of the hall, which was to be our bedroom. We were quite happy to sleep at floor level.

In the morning, after breakfast, we were given our two pence pocket money (now equivalent to less than 1p). The older ones could venture towards the seafront about half a mile away, with instructions to be back for dinner at 12.30 pm and not to swim in the sea or baths.

On two afternoons, the boys who were in the band had to play in the pavilion on the seafront. This used to bring in money, which was given to us all as extra pocket money each day. One day I, and some of the other boys of the choir, sang with the band.

With the holidays over, I returned to school for my last term. Everything was going fine, then – two weeks before I was due to leave – I had an accident at No 16. I was washing up the tea-time things, when it was pointed out to me that the kitchen window was open and had to be shut. I could not reach it, so I climbed up and stood in the sink. The top window was the sash cord type and stiff, so I gave it an extra strong push. The window flew up, I lost my balance, and went backwards from the sink – hitting my head on the tiled floor. I ended up in the infirmary with concussion and bruises for three weeks, so I missed the school leaving ceremony.

Now I thought I would be leaving Erdington, but it was not to be. At 9.00 each morning I had to work in the boot repairing shop. At first I was stripping the old soles and heels off the shoes. The boot repairer, Mr Pollard, would check the shoes and then put on the new leather soles and rubber heels. He was a jolly man, always joking and talking about sport – mainly golf, which I did not know anything about.

After two weeks, he started to show me how to put on soles. He would put the first few nails in, cut around the shoe and remove the overhang of leather, then pencil a line on the edge for me to put the nails in – picking up one at a time.

"Now look. This is the way to do it: put a few sprigs into your hand and tip them in your mouth, then get one ready with your tongue while you knock in a nail."

I tried it, and was just getting the idea with about two or three nails in my mouth, when he patted me on the back, saying, "I think we may make a cobbler of you yet." Down went the nails. He laughed and said, "You'll be alright after Mother Griffiths' jalap."

The afternoons were spent doing jobs in the office, but every Tuesday – at 2.00 pm – I had to take a sterilizing drum from the infirmary to the dispensary at Erdington House, which was on the other side of the road from the homes. I also had to collect it the following day. On one occasion, after taking the drum, I was walking back from the dispensary while a male nurse was walking some of the mentally handicapped children from the hospital. He looked at me and shouted, "Come here!" I ran like hell, in case he gathered me into his group!

On other occasions I had to collect small, sealed containers of swabs from Sister Wilson, which I then had to take to a laboratory at Dudley Road Hospital. I was given the full tram fare and was told to bring the tickets back. I always picked up adult tickets from the trams to hand in when I returned, despite having paid child's fare.

A few days before Christmas, a few of us choirboys would go into the village – past the Abbey, going towards Sutton. There were a number of large Georgian houses, where we had been invited to sing carols for the owners and their guests. We did well out of it, with mince pies and other treats.

8

Outside the Iron Gates

ON FRIDAY 30TH JANUARY 1935, both Norman Hardwicke and I were fitted out with two long-trousered suits, two pairs of shoes, three shirts, ties, pyjamas, underwear, socks, hairbrush, toothbrush and a large expanding case. We dressed and packed all the other items into the suitcase. At 14 years old, I looked – and felt – smart in my first long trouser suit, which fitted me perfectly.

The secretary of the Cottage Homes, Mr Hockaday, came to take us to the working boys' home. He gave us each a Bible and Prayer Book (I still have both today). We walked down the drive, through the Iron Gates with our cases, and on to Gravelly Hill Station – taking a short ride to Vauxhall and Duddeston Station. It was then just a short walk to the working boys' home in Vauxhall Road – a very large house, opposite Great Brook Street. We were met by the superintendent, Mr Squires, who straightaway took us into the washroom and allocated us each a locker. He also took us upstairs and gave us places in one of the four dormitories. We soon settled into the routine, having been told the general rules and that certain duties would be expected and done on a rota. Mr Squires was an ex-naval man and ran the place with the discipline of a ship: strict, but fair.

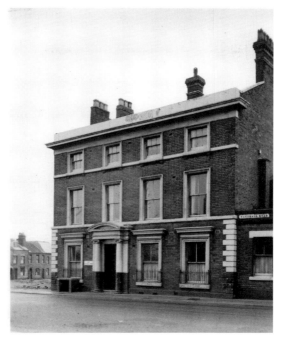

Working boys' home, 205 Vauxhall Rd, Birmingham.
(Birmingham Lives Archive)

The following day I started work as an assembler at a factory (in Chester Street, Aston) making fuse boxes. It was boring and repetitive work. It was a dirty place, which I stuck with for about six months. It was then that I knew that my short stature was of amusement to others, as I was called all sorts of names: Dwarf, Shortie, Midget, Tiny, Short-arse, and many more. At first I used to get mad and bad tempered about it, but later I learnt to ignore it. Then one day I collected my wages, told the foreman I was not coming back, and I walked out. I told Mr Squires that I had been sacked, to which he replied, "You had better get out in the morning and find another job quickly."

9

From Electric to Gas

THE NEXT MORNING I just wandered around, then found myself near Stechford Station – walking down the hill. On the right was a large works. When I got to the bottom, I bucked up courage and asked at the gatehouse if there were any jobs.
"Yes Sonny, if you go up to the new assembly shop and ask for Mr Starkey." In those days, the foreman was the hire and fire man. When he saw me, he said – with a smile on his face – "Come and try again when you have grown a bit more, Sonny."

Whilst walking away from the assembly department, a man stopped me and asked what I was doing inside the works. I replied that I had been after a job and told him the response of the foreman. He took me back to the department and spoke to the foreman, pointing out a youth (who was 6 ft. tall) bending down to fit legs to gas stoves. He told the foreman to "Get that guy on a job to suit his height", to put "this little fellow" on the job, and if "he" was not satisfactory after two weeks then to "kick his bloody arse out of it". (It was later that I found out that the man was a management advisor.)

I got on with the job, along with the additional job of teaboy for the department. This was quite lucrative and it gave me as much money in tips as my wages: in those days, ten shillings (50p) per week of 49 hours. About three weeks later, the foreman said, "I want you in the office." I thought my time had come. He asked where I lived. I told him it was 205 Vauxhall Road.

"Now look here Laddie, I have just had your boss inquiring about how you are getting along and also saying that you are from a working boys' home. So once again, what is your address, as I don't like people who tell lies?"

I replied that I did not tell lies, that I did live at 205 Vauxhall Road – which was the number of the house – and that I did not have to say it was a boys' home. After all, I had not done anything wrong. He replied, "All right, get back to work." I thought that was the end of the matter, but oh no – someone else in the office had overheard the conversation.

I wondered why, all of a sudden, for the next few days I was being avoided by the rest of the workers. Some were asking what I had done wrong and why I was in a home. This continued and I got bad tempered about it. Then one of the older men took me to one side during lunch-time and talked to me about my being aggressive to the others. I told him a little of my life and the reason for being in the homes. He said, "Leave it with me Son; I will soon put things right." He left me and went straight in to the foreman, and a few of the boys and men were given a dressing down. Things then got a lot better, as they started to accept me for who I was.

A few days later, the foreman was having a heated argument with one of the men and called me over.

"What's this I hear? You won't make this man's tea or get him his sandwiches from the canteen?"

"All the other men give me a penny or twopence a week for doing it, but he doesn't give me anything, so I stopped," I snapped back.

"Good for you, Boy," replied the foreman, and he really got stuck into the other worker.

After a few months, I requested the chance to do other work in the assembly of gas stoves. Often this meant standing on a box to reach. Later I moved on to benchwork, again needing to stand on a box to do filing of cast iron parts, pipe bending and threading, etc.

One day, the works manager was showing a party around the works. On reaching where I was working, he remarked to the people, "We even have people made to measure for the job", which amused them. But I responded very quickly for all to hear, "It would be far better if the bench was made to measure." Within half an hour, the carpenter was in the department reducing the height of the bench to suit me. That bench moved with me to various departments, as I changed jobs.

The routine at the home was quite reasonable. After getting away from work and having tea, we were able to go out, but had to be in by 9.00 pm – except for Saturday, when it was 9.30 pm.

I soon found out the dodge at the Ashted Cinema. The price of going in was 3d, so it was arranged that one lad would pay to get in. He would then go to the gents', which was near an exit, and would open the push bar door at the side and let two others in – so it only cost us 1d each!

Saturday lunchtime was when pocket money was handed out by Mr Squires. You had to take with you one pair of socks, washed and darned, which he would check. He would then hand out pocket money for the week: one penny for each shilling earned, plus sixpence. That meant that, for my ten shillings a week, I received one shilling and fourpence (approximately 7p).

Some nights we would walk into town and go to the Bull Ring. It used to be great fun to hear the religious speakers and also the jockeys trying to sell tips. But best of all was the man who was in a straitjacket and chained up; after rolling about, he always got free inside the three minutes allotted time.

Occasionally, on Saturday afternoons, we would join the queue for the first house at the Hippodrome; sometimes waiting about two hours. For sixpence (just over 2p), and dashing up the stairs, you might be lucky to get a seat (the three back rows only). Otherwise, you had to stand at the back for the whole show. We saw wonderful shows, with stars like Stainless Stephen, Max Miller, Wilson Keppel and Betty, Ann Ziegler and Webster Booth, and "Hutch" (Leslie Hutchison).

If you did not want to go out, then down the garden was a half-sized billiards table and also a large hut where you could play table tennis. The trouble was that when I played billiards – which I enjoyed – I had to use the rest most of the time because I just could not reach when the ball was away from the cushion.

In March 1937, as my wages were now 18 shillings per week (90p), Mr Squires said that I was now able to look after myself and should go into lodgings.

10

Out to the Wide World

MR SQUIRES INTRODUCED me to a couple named Mr and Mrs Aplin, who lived at Kenelm Road, Small Heath. I went to their place and settled in. They had a son, who was 18 years old, and we got along fine. Money was hard going for a time, as my eighteen shillings (90p) was split into fourteen shillings (70p) for board and lodgings, and two shillings (10p) for bus and tram fares to get to work. This left me with two shillings (10p) for pocket money, and I had to buy clothes and odd items out of that.

As time went by, the Aplins moved to a new house in Gleneagles Road, Yardley. I went with them and things were getting better. I still had to report to the Working Boys' Home once a month, then one day Mr Squires told me that, as I was doing well, I need not go again. He gave me £1-2-0 (one pound and two shillings, equivalent to £1.10 today) which was still in my clothing account. He told me to put it in the bank and said that he would like me to return for the last time, showing him the bank book with it in. This I did the following week.

Things were going fine. I needed a new suit and went into town to 'Weaver and Weaver' tailors, where I was measured for a suit costing thirty shillings (£1.50). It was a beautiful brown serge suit and I looked smart. I was also given a free pair of shoes with it. Three days later I received a voucher for five shillings (25p) off the next made-to-measure suit – what a bargain!

Now I was able to go anywhere I liked, I went across town to the Middlemore Homes in Weoley Park and asked if I could see my brother, Ken (who was then 11 years old). The Matron there said "Of course", and Ken joined me in the reception room. He was just a little taller than me. While we talked about the place and how he was doing at school, a lady came in with a tray of tea and biscuits. When she left, Ken said, "You had better come more often!" He told me that he would not be going overseas as he was medically unsuitable, and that he would be going to Kings Norton Grammar School soon. I thought about how lucky he was. On leaving, I told him that I would do my best to see him about every 2 months, which I did.

Then times were getting a little uncertain. There was talk of war. Mrs Aplin's son had to register for the militia, which called up 20-year-olds to train for the armed forces. Then on 1st September 1939 – my 19th birthday – we learned, during the morning at work, that Germany had moved into Poland. During the day, several of the workers in the factory were called out to report to various barracks etc.

On Saturday 2nd September, an air raid shelter was delivered to every house in Gleneagles Road. Sunday was a brilliant day, sun shining, with the prospect of it being very hot. Early after breakfast, Mr Aplin and I went to the bottom of the garden and started to dig. It was decided to combine next door's shelter with ours. This meant that we had to dig a hole 16 feet, by 6 feet, by 4 feet deep. Part way through the job, we stopped; partly for tea and a rest, but more importantly to listen to the Prime Minister, Mr Chamberlain, speak at 11 o'clock to tell us that we were at war with Germany. More determined to get on with the job, I went out again – shirt off. We really got stuck in and the sun was now getting hot.

After Sunday lunch, we went back again. Then, just before tea, we started to put the pieces of arched corrugated iron into the hole and bolted them together. After tea, we finally finished it off by covering the top and sides with the soil that we had taken from the hole. Feeling proud of our day's work, I went and had a bath to remove the dirt and sweat of the day. I then realised that the sun had done its worst to my back, chest and arms. I blistered – the pain was awful for days.

Three weeks later, although we had had hardly any rain, the shelter had 3 feet of water inside – so had most of the others in the road. After a period of time, the local authority concreted the bottom and sides to ground level: this cured the problem. Thankfully we had had no reason to use it at that time.

Early in November the calling up age was reduced to 19 years, so I had to register. I was ragged and called all sorts of names by the others in the queue at the local labour exchange. Late in December, I received my papers to present myself for medical examination at the Albert Hall, Victoria Road, Aston. On the request was printed "Fleet Air Arm (Flying Duties)."

I attended, as stated. When I went in, the orderly took me into the hall. I filled in the form with name, address, etc, then moved on to where the doctors were checking. I was told to stand on the scales; they just checked my height and told me I need not bother to undress, but just to move along in turn to each doctor. All the others were stripped. Each doctor signed the forms and moved me on. At the end of it all, I was told that I would be hearing in a few days time. A week later, I received a letter from Ernest Bevin (Minister of Labour) stating that I was declared unsuitable on medical grounds for the armed forces, but that I could be used on important war work. I was to report to Birmingham Central Labour Exchange, where I would be directed to vital work – even if it meant being in another part of the country.

I went along and gave the paper to the official at the counter.

"Yes," he said, "where are you working at present?"

I replied, "Parkinson Stove Co."

"You can't leave there, they are on 100% war work."

I laughed at him and said, "Do you call making gas stoves 'war work'?"

"Just a minute, I will check," he said. Then he came back and said, "Yes, we know, but you will not be allowed to move."

So there I stayed. I was asked at the works if I would join the gas disposal squad. I was trained on gas detection, how to treat victims, and clearing and cleansing contaminated areas. Thankfully we were never put to the test.

At home I joined the civil defence as an air raid warden, with duties in the road and at the control post (which was at Cockshut Hill School, where we had a room behind the stage in the main hall). On Saturday evenings there were dances and I would always watch. I wished I could learn to dance, but I was not plucky enough.

Then I found out that the works had started having dancing lessons in the canteen, one night per week. I went along, just because a few of my fellow-workers were having fun at my expense – talking about how they would like to see "Shortie Mackenzie" dancing with the girls. The dancing teacher looked at me, amazed, then said, "If you have had the guts to come, I promise you will dance in time." He told the women who were there that if they refused to dance with anyone, then he would not allow them at future classes. After a few months I was getting confident, so I started going to dances when able.

The air raids were on. After I had been at work all day, got home and had my evening meal, off would go the siren. This meant I had to go over to the ARP (Air Raid Precautions) post for instructions of areas to be covered. We did get a couple of houses destroyed by bombs in the early part of the war. Later the main problem was incendiary bombs, which were dealt with mainly by smothering with sandbags. On one occasion a fire bomb dropped into a house over the road. When I was let into the house, I dashed upstairs into the bedroom: an incendiary was burning on top of the bed. I opened the window, gathered the bedclothes, and threw the lot out. The woman was not pleased – she said that I should not have thrown out the bedclothes, only the small bomb. She did not realise that her whole house could have burned!

One night I went into town, to the Odeon Cinema in New Street, Birmingham. At about 8.30pm, the warning of an air raid was flashed on the screen. When the film finished we were told to stay where we were, as it would not have been wise to go outside and no transport was getting into the city centre. I did try to leave, but the police made me stay – although I had told them I would be expected at an ARP post. The organist played for a while, then people got up on the stage and entertained the audience. It was amazing the talent these people had and the wonderful spirit of those times.

When we were eventually allowed out – at 6.00am – the area around New Street, High Street, and the Bull Ring was devastated, with plenty of fires. On the way home, I was told that a bomb had fallen in Weoley Park Road. So after getting home and having something to eat, I was out again. I was anxious to find out if my brother was all right – the Middlemore Homes were in Weoley Park Road. The bus into town had to take a lot of diversions, because of bomb damage and fires which were still burning.

I got a tramcar at Navigation Street. It got as far as Sun Street when we all had to get off and walk about half a mile to the next tram, as the lines were broken near a large crater in the road. While walking along Bristol Road, I heard a tune coming from a house which had suffered damage. It was a wonderful sound: I stopped and listened. It just did not add up, such beautiful music in a devastated area. I was haunted by that tune for months, then I found out that it was Tchaikovsky's 'Serenade for Strings'. I still love to hear that piece of music today.

I got to the Middlemore Homes in Weoley Park Road to find that my brother had been evacuated to Gloucester with his school, Kings Norton Grammar, a few weeks earlier.

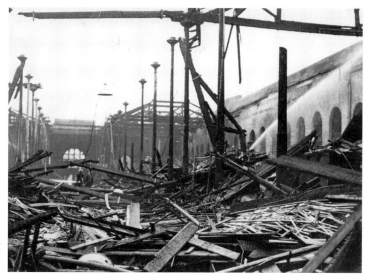

Birmingham's Bull Ring markets, following an air raid in August 1940.
(Birmingham Lives Archive)

The people at that time were wonderful. Everyone helped each other and was friendly, even in difficult times.

As time went on, I was getting the odd letter from my sister, Betty. One day I had a letter from her, stamped on the envelope "Opened by Censor". When I opened it, the two pages were nothing but a lot of slotted holes: it appeared that she had met a number of navy men from the Birmingham area while they were in Perth and Geraldton (Western Australia) and wanted me to pass on some messages to their relatives. But I could not make top nor tail out of it all. I often wondered what tune would have come out if I had put the letter in a pianola!

I had another letter from my brother Ken, telling me that he had joined the army. He had got into trouble as he had said he was 18 years old, but when questioned about why he had not registered for that age group – and after a lot of checking on his true age (17 years) – he was allowed to stay.

When he had his leave, he used to stay with me at my digs and was welcomed by Mrs Aplin. I was surprised to find that he had rapidly grown to six feet tall.

Ken was always the joker. On one occasion I had just bought a pair of shoes and, having got home, put them down in the hall. Mrs Aplin asked where they were, so I went into the hall and took the bag into the living room. When I pulled out the box and opened it, there was only one shoe inside – I was amazed. Ken said that I must have left it at the shop. So I put the shoe back into the box, put on my coat, and said that I would see them all later. I had gone down the road with the bag – and was about to get on the bus – when Ken dashed up, saying they had found the other shoe. He had taken it out when I had arrived home!

On another occasion, when Ken was on leave, my girlfriend (Zeta) and I had bought some wool (as she had promised to knit me a Fair Isle pullover). So I had to hold the wool, while she wound it into balls. Suddenly she said, "I am sure we have wound up more than we bought." Then we realised that Ken and Mrs Aplin had undone the balls of wool and rewound them into skeins. Was she mad!

11

Mother's Death

I RECEIVED A LETTER from Australia, in which my sister, Betty, informed me that she had been told that our mother had died twelve months previously. The letter had taken seven months to get to me, so actually we were looking at between 18 months and 2 years after my mother's death. I was more in a temper than upset, so I told Mrs Aplin that in the morning I would be off to York.

I was at New Street bright and early to catch the train. This time I soon sorted out the new address, which was in Boroughbridge Road. When I arrived at the house, at about 12.30 pm, the door was opened by a man, who looked at me and said, "Is it Bob?" He said that he was Uncle Bert.

"Come on in, your aunt will not be very long coming from church."

I told him why I was there and that I wanted to know why I had not been told about my mother.

"Wait until everyone is here and we shall discuss it after dinner. You will have dinner with us? There is plenty."

Aunt Jennie arrived from church with her 17-year-old daughter, Eileen. This was the first time that I had seen Eileen. After being introduced, they went into the kitchen.

After a short time, Eileen was setting the table and the meal was soon ready. The starter was individual Yorkshire puddings with gravy. Then, using the same plate, the small roast was carved and we helped ourselves to potatoes and carrots. When all was cleared away and washed up, we then started to talk. I was getting a little hot-tempered, so Aunt Jennie told me to calm down. She explained, telling me that my mother had been in hospital as a patient for some time and was unable to write. Therefore I had not written to her, so Aunt Jennie could not find out my address. But she did find a letter from Betty, so informed her. She said that she was sorry, but what else could she do?

The subject was changed: we discussed the time I had come to York over 10 years earlier. It was then that I found out that Mother had been at the house. They said that they had kept her indoors because they thought that my father was setting a trap.

Later, during the evening, I left and returned to Brum[4] – with an invitation to spend a long weekend with them in a month's time. This I accepted and when I did go back I had a wonderful time. I was grateful that we were able to understand each other's point of view, with no bad feelings.

---

4 Birmingham

12

Betty Returns to England

IN FEBRUARY 1948 I received a letter from my sister Betty, telling me she was returning to England. She was taking the opportunity to accompany two elderly ladies as nurse/companion for the boat journey. I got in touch with Ken, so we could both arrange our holidays to fit with her arrival in early May. The plan was for Betty to settle the two elderly ladies first, then make her own way to Birmingham from London.

The day arrived when she was due in Birmingham. Ken came from his place in Thornton Heath, Surrey, arriving mid-morning. After a long discussion, as we did not know which London station she would be coming from, we agreed that Ken would go to Snow Hill Station and I would go to New Street Station. We went off to town at about 2.00pm and split to our respective stations.

I stood on the steps leading down to Platform 2 and saw several trains in from London, but no sign of Betty. Just after 6.30pm I went across to Snow Hill and saw Ken, who was also becoming a bit concerned; however we decided to wait at our stations until 9.30pm. So I was back at New Street when, at about 8.00pm, Mrs Aplin's son came dashing over to me saying that Betty was at home! We went over to Snow Hill, met Ken, then travelled back to Gleneagles Road where Betty was well settled in.

It was quite an emotional moment, the first time we had been together for fifteen years, and we were in tears.

Betty told us about her arrival at New Street Station, with her luggage, which comprised of two cabin trunks and two large suitcases. She had got a porter and had been taken through the tunnel under the railway lines to get a taxi, and then on to Gleneagles Road. During our rather late evening meal, Betty told us of her journey from London, saying she was most impressed at the countryside and was amazed at the number of greens she had noticed in the trees, hedgerows and fields.

The next morning, after breakfast, Betty said that she would like to go across to the Middlemore Homes, so all three of us went. On arrival, we asked to see the superintendent. We were welcomed into his office and he said how pleased he was to see Betty and Ken. He asked Betty how she had found Australia, and had she any comments on Fairbridge Farm School? She replied, rather sharply, that she thought it was wrong that the children out there were expected to go about in bare feet all the time. When the time came for them to leave and to work on farms or in industry, or for girls to go into domestic service, putting on boots or shoes became quite an ordeal.

Having got that off her chest, the discussion turned to what Betty was going to do now, as she had returned permanently. At this stage the matron joined us and suggested Betty go for a nursing appointment, as she was qualified in Australia. Betty said she would prefer childcare, as she wished to add to her general nursing and midwifery. The superintendent immediately got on the phone and arranged for her to be considered for a post at a small children's home in Yardley, which accommodated around twelve young children and which would be a living in post. It was settled and arranged that she would start in a week's time.

During the next few days we took Betty around Birmingham to acclimatise her with the local surroundings. On one occasion we called into a local pub and, over drinks, we discussed our respective lives. What had we achieved and how had we overcome the various problems we had encountered? Would it have been better if the happenings of the past had been different?

We came to the conclusion that we were lucky to have lived and to have overcome the problems we had experienced, which were not of our making. We then came to the question of what we would have done if our parents had turned up. I was asked to be honest and to say what I would have done in this situation. My reply was that I would always respect and welcome my mother, but as for my father, I would ignore him completely. After all, he had got rid of me by sending me off to York!

Betty's response was just the opposite, saying she would welcome Father but could not reconcile with Mother – as she had broken up the family and was responsible for Betty being sent to Australia. Ken was blunt and bitter about the whole affair, saying he would not acknowledge either and adding "Why should we bother?", as we had made our own way in life with a certain amount of success without them. Although we differed, we respected each others' points of view.

Betty started work at the children's home and would occasionally come across to see me at my digs. After about four months, she told me she had been applying for other posts around the country and had been successful at a place in

Yorkshire. She would be moving the following week. She was there for a few weeks and moved on again, several times. I discussed it with Ken when he came to see me. We came to the conclusion that she was not at all happy living in England and would not settle. So it came as no surprise to hear from her that she had been in touch with the Middlemore Homes and had arranged for a return to Australia. She would be in charge of a party of children being sent out there, which meant she was being paid and also had a free passage. She also requested that Ken and I were not to make arrangements to see her off. In any case we did not know when, or from which port, they would be going. I did go across to the Middlemore Homes to find out, but to no avail – they said that all information was confidential.

So we did not hear from Betty until she arrived in Fremantle, Western Australia. She returned to nursing in Kalamunda and we kept in touch by monthly letters. She was certainly much happier over there and became an Australian citizen.

13

A Little Stagestruck

WHEN THE WAR with Germany was over, there had been a relaxation of war work and the company went back to its normal work (of making gas cookers and fires). It was then that I realised that I needed to do something, as the whole approach to work – and to methods of production – was changing fast. So I went to night school at Birmingham Technical College and studied in the Department of Industrial Administration. The subjects covered were: personnel management, factory organisation, works safety, costing and estimating, industrial law, etc. All of these I found stimulating, and very useful when at a later time I was able to take my first steps into junior management.

When I returned to work after the annual holiday in August 1949, the personnel director sent for me. He began talking about the company and its future, then asked how I spent my hours away from the factory. I told him that my main leisure activity was ballroom dancing and that I was also doing three nights a week at technical college. It was then that he butted in, saying that he had undertaken to produce the next play to be put on by the company's drama group, the 'Parkinson Players'. He added that it was an unusual type of venture for amateur dramatics, as it would be in the true tradition of the Chinese theatre. This, he explained, meant that the whole play is performed on a stage without the scenery that is normally used in British and American productions.

I felt that the director was trying to get me interested, but to what purpose? With a smile on his face he said that he would like to see me join the group, adding that he was discussing this venture with a number of employees, from management, office staff and the shop floor. He pointed out that, if he could get a good mix of employees, it would be helpful in improving industrial relations. He hoped that we could all pull together and that our respective positions at work would be forgotten.

A week later the personnel director called a meeting of all the people he had spoken to. With about sixty at the gathering, he told us that the proposed venture was a production of 'Lady Precious Stream' by S. I. Hsiung and that he would be needing 35-40 in the cast. He also required a stage manager and other backstage workers. At the next meeting, he started his selection of the cast. I was requested to partner a six-foot colleague to play the comedy roles, as 'Equerries to the Princess'.

During the following six weeks we attended rehearsals two nights a week; reading, learning the lines, and getting the feel of the story. By the second week of November we were gradually getting it together – it was great fun! The play was to be produced at the Bottville Hall, Acocks Green, which had a very good stage and could seat about 400. The two Sundays before we were due to put it on, we all gathered at the works social club (which had a small stage) to have a full rehearsal. We went through the play twice on each occasion.

On December 6th, at the end of the day's work, we all met in the canteen at 5.30pm and were provided with tea and sand-wiches. Then, in one of the company's covered lorries, we moved to Acocks Green to give a full dress rehearsal to an invited audience of local pensioners. It was well received by the gathering, which gave us satisfaction and encouragement. The next two nights it was for real – we were playing to the paying public.

It went off well and the audience were very appreciative of our efforts. Of course there were roars of laughter every time I appeared with my six-foot partner as Ma Ta and Kiang Hai ("the long and the short"). It was a very ambitious venture, which proved to be successful. The following evening we gathered in the social club for a party given by the directors.

After the success of 'Lady Precious Stream', the Players were called to another meeting, in January 1950, to discuss the next production. It was decided to go for a comedy and we eventually selected 'The Blue Goose' by Peter Blakemore. Immediately the newly-appointed producer got down to choosing his cast and I was amazed to find I had been selected for a principal role, as 'The Mayor'.

During the rehearsals, the lady responsible for costumes took just four measurements of me (height, chest, inside leg and length of arm), saying she was sending off to Moss Bros for the hire of formal evening dress for some of the male characters. When dressed with white tie and tails at the dress rehearsal, again for an invited audience of local pensioners, I really looked smart and distinguished. We played for three nights, each with a full house and roars of laughter from the audience – the Parkinson Players had achieved another success!

Later we prepared for yet another play, 'The Warrior's Husband' by Julian Thompson. This time I was appointed stage manager, which I found most interesting and rewarding. It was again a most successful effort by all the cast.

It was at this stage in my life that I felt everything was coming my way, with many friends. I also took up other activities: ice skating and horse riding. One Sunday, a few of us at the stables went riding to the Clent Hills. We would be away about four or five hours, stopping somewhere for light refreshments and leaving the horses in the adjoining yard. I popped to the toilet and, when I returned to join the others outside, they were all gone with their horses – leaving just my horse, which I could not mount. So I just led the horse and walked a little way. Then I found the others round the corner, enjoying the fun!

14

Marjorie

THE WORKS DANCING CLASSES resumed in late 1951 with a different teacher, Dick Holloway. After a few weeks he asked me if I would go to his place in Horrell Road, Sheldon, where he had a dancing studio at the rear of his house and was short of men in his classes. So I bucked up courage and went along, mainly just to see what it was like. The studio was at the bottom of his garden; he had built it himself. It was about fifty foot square, with a proper dance floor of maple and also an excellent record player with plenty of Victor Sylvester records. I danced with the ladies who were there and in particular with Marjorie, who was about the same age as myself (I was 31). She appeared to be a bit snooty and looked down on me, and not because she was slightly taller than me. A few weeks later we had a works dance and I asked Marjorie if she would like to come along. "Yes," was her reply, only because she found out some of the other women were going and also Dick Holloway, the dance instructor.

I used to walk Marjorie part of the way home from dance classes, and then it became a little further, until eventually I walked her to her door. Then I was asked if I would like to call in for supper one night the next week, which I accepted. When I arrived on the evening in question, I was surprised to find that all Marjorie's family were there and the table was well laid, with plenty of food. I wondered whether they were curious about me, or my size, but as the evening wore on I was chatty and all went well. The family appeared to

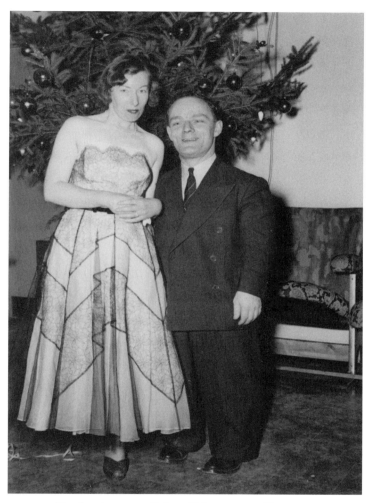

The dancing years: Bob and Marjorie at a Christmas
dance in the 1950s. Bob was a keen dancer (he had several
dancing medals) and had met Marjorie at dance classes.
(Photograph courtesy of Sharon Wiltshire)

have forgotten my height – in fact, it was a very enjoyable evening.

At about the same time, a weekend social trip to Paris was being planned at the works – following the success of a day trip to Amsterdam the previous year. Marjorie heard about it from another source and asked if she could come along, so I booked her a place. The morning of May 10th 1952 was bright and sunny. I met Marjorie and we were picked up by coach and taken to Elmdon Aerodrome (now Birmingham Airport), where we all boarded the waiting plane. There was an air of excitement as we rose from the runway. About thirty minutes into the flight someone shouted that we were crossing the coast and to look down – there was Brighton Pier. Marjorie looked out and when she saw the sea she felt sick, wondering if she would survive the rest of the flight!

Arriving at Le Bourget airfield we were met by our courier, who escorted us to the coach and then on to the hotel in the Rue de Provence, where we had lunch. The afternoon was free for sampling the shops, but prices were beyond our limited currency allowance, which was £15 for the weekend. Marjorie and I walked along the Champs Élysées, window shopping, but she was very disappointed, expecting to see plenty of young ladies showing off the latest fashion. In fact, she thought they were dressed rather drably. The traffic was amazing; they all seemed to be in a hurry, sounding their horns at the slightest hold-up. We thought they were all mad!

Back at the hotel we tidied up for dinner in the restaurant, after which we were taken by coach for a tour of the city with all the prominent places floodlit. It was a wonderful sight. Then we were taken to the Moulin Rouge and shown to our reserved tables on a small balcony. We had a light meal and champagne while watching the excellent floorshow, which finished in a boisterous mood with the can-can – as only they know how!

Next morning after breakfast, which was just bread rolls and coffee, we toured the city. At the Arc de Triomphe we stood silent for a while at the tomb of 'le Soldat Inconnu' with its perpetual flame, then went by lift to the top and saw a most impressive view of Paris with its wide boulevards branching out. We visited Napoleon's tomb and later Notre-Dame Cathedral, where we were able to go round even though a service was in progress. It was now midday, so we returned to the hotel for lunch; after which we collected our belongings, as the afternoon was to be spent at the Palais de Versailles before our return to England.

We were given a comprehensive tour of the palace, seeing the beautiful painted ceilings, statues and galleries of paintings, and also the famous Hall of Mirrors. The gardens were spacious and elegant. We were able to wander and spend time admiring the beauty of it all, before returning to the coach which took us to Le Bourget for our return home.

It was a crowded and memorable weekend, which I enjoyed and so did Marjorie in the end – after her unfortunate bout of sickness earlier. And all at the cost of twelve guineas (£12.60) each!

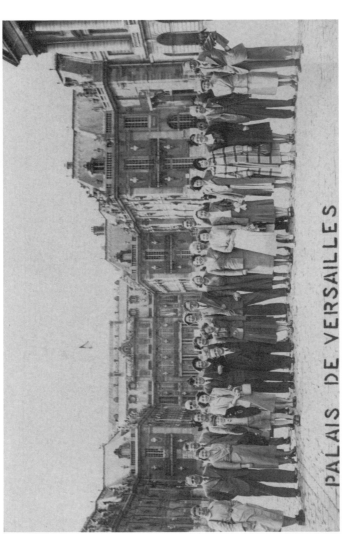

At the Palais de Versailles during the Parkinson Cowan Social Club weekend in Paris, 1952. Bob is in the front row (to the left of centre) with Marjorie beside him.

(Photograph courtesy of Sharon Wiltshire)

15

Decisions

THE NEXT MONTH, in June 1952, I was amazed to be called to attend a management meeting. I must admit that I was a little concerned about what it was all about and wondered, 'Why me?'

It was quite a shock when the sales director said that he would like me to consider a change of job. He wanted me to take on the opening of a repair section, adding that there would be times when I would have to travel to gas board depots around the country to do repairs and adjustments, some of which might need to be done in the customer's home. It would mean some days and nights away from the works and home, for which I would get expenses and travel vouchers. He added that I had been selected by the management team for my knowledge of the company and its products. So when asked if I was interested, I jumped at the chance. I saw it as an opportunity to progress and get away from the assembly lines.

My first venture was to North Thames Gas Board, in Fulham, London. I did wonder how I would be received by them, but when they realised my capabilities they forgot my height – so all was well and I certainly felt a lot better.

I also became involved with the company's new models at the pre-production stage. One model in particular was a whole new concept in gas cookers, with eye-level grill and flash ignition to all burners (including oven and grill) from one

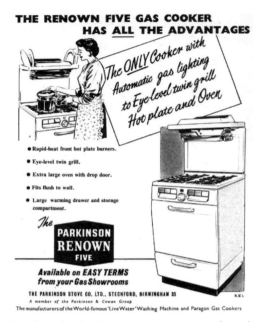

An advert for the Parkinson Renown Five (1955).
(Reproduced with the permission of Electrolux plc)

central pilot light. It was going to be called the 'Coronation' but for some reason this was changed to 'Renown Five' when it went on the assembly line. It was practically hand-built due to parts not fitting correctly!

Away from work, Marjorie and I were getting along fine, going to many dances and the cinema. In fact, it was becoming serious. That made me think, 'Where was I going?' I gave a lot of thought to it and decided I would make an appointment to see my doctor. I told him that I was friendly with a very nice young lady and it was becoming serious. I asked him to be honest and frank: was my problem of height of a hereditary nature? He said that he would look into it, but asked if I would wait until he had cleared his surgery. I waited for just over an hour; it was 9.00pm when he called me in. Just as we were about to start talking, his wife brought in a tray of tea and sandwiches for both of us. After a lot of questions, which I answered to the best of my knowledge, he got out a number of books and read quite a lot of passages on cases of Achondroplasia[5].

It was after 11.30pm when he said that, in his opinion, there was little to worry about as Marjorie was of near normal height. Had she been of the same condition as me it might have been a different matter, but his advice was to go ahead. "Good luck to you both", he said. I thanked him for his time and patience. As I was walking home, feeling quite perked up, Yardley Church clock struck midnight.

A week later I proposed to Marjorie. She accepted and we were engaged on her birthday, 29th November 1952. Then we started preparing for the wedding. After a lot of discussion, we decided it would be 29th August 1953.

Mrs Aplin, my landlady, who was now widowed, wanted me to stay with her and offered me two rooms. I said I was sorry, but that I wanted to start off by getting a place of our own. Marjorie and I spent a few weekends looking at building sites, with a view to buying a house. We eventually found a site at Bacons End, near Coleshill. No houses had been built, but we liked the area so I paid a deposit and staked my claim.

---

[5] Achondroplasia is a rare genetic condition that affects a single gene called FGFR3, resulting in abnormal cartilage formation. A person with achondroplasia can pass the condition on to his or her children. If one parent is affected by achondroplasia and the other is not, their children have a 50% chance of being born with the condition. This is because achondroplasia is an example of a 'dominant' genetic condition.

I told Marjorie's mother of our choice and she went into the kitchen, where I heard her telling the others, "He is buying a house." Giving the impression that I was very well off.

The wedding took place at Yardley Parish Church. After the ceremony and party, my brother drove us to the station. When we settled in our seats for the journey to Hastings, he showered us with loads of confetti – much to the amusement of the other passengers in the compartment! Not having told anyone where we would be staying, it came as a shock when the landlady announced at breakfast, "Welcome to the newly-weds, Bob and Marjorie Mackenzie!"

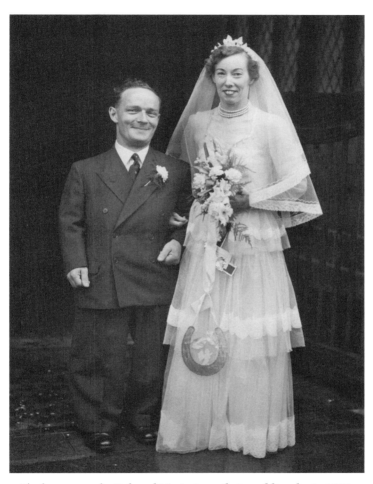

The happy couple: Bob and Marjorie on their wedding day in 1953.
They were happily married until Marjorie's death in 2001.
(Photograph courtesy of Sharon Wiltshire)

16

Conclusion

(Written in 1996)

HAVING SURVIVED 75 years, I have no regrets. What I went through in my early years taught me tolerance, understanding, and that you only get out of life what you yourself are prepared to put into it.

In my case, it was always to try and do all things better than the other guy and, even if it meant time and money for training and tuition, to achieve my aims in life. Also, I found if you allow others to see that you are capable, they will accept and respect you for it.

So my advice to all small people is to work hard and try to do what is best for you, just that little better. It will pay off and I know it can be done. Good luck to you all!

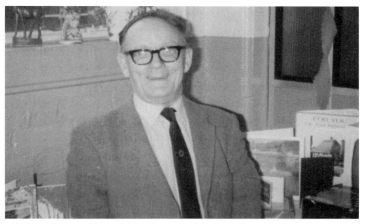

End of an era: Bob on the day he retired from Parkinson Cowan in 1983, after more than 40 years of working for the company. During his long retirement, Bob took up writing and recorded his life story.

(Photograph courtesy of Sharon Wiltshire)

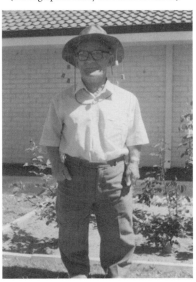

Happier days: Bob visiting his sister in Australia in 1985. Despite being on opposite sides of the world, Bob and Betty remained close until her death in 1993.

(Photograph courtesy of Sharon Wiltshire)